D1572265

Fibromyalgia

A Guide to the Symptoms, Management, and Treatment of Fibromyalgia and Chronic Fatigue

Jessica Rose

Table of Contents

Introduction

Thank you for choosing this book! Whether you have fibromyalgia or are just looking to understand better what fibromyalgia is, this book will be able to help. The more you know about fibromyalgia, the easier it will be for you to help yourself or a loved one deal with this challenging condition. So much is currently unknown about fibromyalgia, but we can use what we do know to promote positive changes in the lives of those who face fibromyalgia every day.

The following chapters will discuss what fibromyalgia is, how it is diagnosed, the symptoms that accompany it, and how it is treated. This book will not just give you the broad strokes of what the condition is, but concisely, it will delve into some of the facets of fibromyalgia that you might not know. It will give you information on the signs and symptoms that you need to know as you are first learning about this condition. It will guide you through the diagnostic process, which will show you how to know if you might have fibromyalgia and how to raise your concerns with your doctor. Moreover, this book will explain to you the different treatment options, both regular and alternative. Finally, it will give you some handy self-help tips for managing fibromyalgia day to day.

Thank you once again for taking the time to read this book. I hope you find it to be both helpful, and informative.

Chapter 1: What Is Fibromyalgia?

Definition

Fibromyalgia, or Fibromyalgia Syndrome (FMS), is a condition that makes people experience chronic pain and fatigue. Being chronic, it is a long-term condition that can impact people throughout their lives. It is a condition that has long been mysterious, but medical professionals are slowly beginning to uncover more and more about what might cause it, and how it can best be treated.

While some people struggle with this condition non-stop, for others, the symptoms can come and go in cycles, and there are some breaks from the constant pain. No one person will entirely represent what fibromyalgia is. The people who experience this disorder are diverse and experience their conditions in ways that are unique to them. If you are a sufferer, a loved one of a sufferer, or if you think you may have this condition, it's essential to know that fibromyalgia impacts so much of the body that it can be hard to pinpoint all the symptoms and to treat the disease directly. Nevertheless, there is hope for people dealing with FMS.

Fibromyalgia can be particularly debilitating because it doesn't just impact one part of the body. People with Fibromyalgia often feel pain all over, which can make it hard to engage in ordinary activities. For people with FMS, it can be hard to find a balance between being too active and being too sedentary, because both can make symptoms worse.

Luckily, fibromyalgia doesn't do any lasting damage to the body. If fibromyalgia causes you to feel pain in your leg, you're not going to do irreparable damage if you walk on that leg. It also doesn't cause any inflammation that you can detect, which separates it from other pain conditions like arthritis (although these conditions can co-occur with fibromyalgia). When you have fibromyalgia, it can be hard for a doctor to see, or detect your pain. It's not like a broken bone that you can see is broken. This makes it hard to diagnose and understand, and it also means that some people don't take it seriously.

FMS symptoms often come and go over time, so people with this condition may get a reprieve from pain occasionally. However, even if you can go a few weeks without significant symptoms, you might have months where your symptoms are severe. The symptoms you have now may also not be the same as the ones you have a year from now.

Causes

Fibromyalgia is a mysterious condition that no one understands fully. Unlike other conditions, we don't have clear definitions and diagnostic criteria to use for diagnosis. The musculoskeletal pain that people with fibromyalgia feel cannot be attributed to any single cause. Several things could potentially cause fibromyalgia, combining together to create the dreadful symptoms that people experience. Medical professionals are still unaware of what the exact causes of this condition are, but they are continuing to complete research to crack the mystery that is fibromyalgia.

Research suggests that people with fibromyalgia follow the multiple-hit theory, which is the idea that there are complicated, multifaceted factors that result in the triggering of fibromyalgia. Thus, this condition probably has hereditary factors and then can be set off by several other factors. Therefore, someone could have genes that predispose them to FMS, but it isn't until they face several triggers that they develop fibromyalgia in the first place. Therefore, a wide range of factors could be causal, and what things trigger one person could be different from what triggers another person. While the exact causes of fibromyalgia are widely unknown, there are some theories about what can make the condition worse.

Doctors have linked genetic factors to FMS. This disorder is potentially the result of gene mutation, and while research is still being done to show a more exact connection, some specific genes seem like they are related to FMS. FMS could potentially occur because these gene mutations affect your body's ability to signal pain correctly. Thus, the nerve cells will be sent signals they aren't supposed to be sent, and you can feel unexplained pain as a result. If you have family members with this condition, you likely have higher odds of having it yourself, so it is worth investigating further with your doctor if you have both a family history of FMS, and widespread pain.

Stress has been shown to have a large influence on FMS. Stressed people are more likely to have heart issues, diabetes, and several other conditions. Thus, it makes sense that stress could be a significant factor in fibromyalgia as well. Stress can also induce hormonal changes that shift how your body reacts and sends signals through your body. As a result, you might develop FMS, and feel pain when you aren't supposed to. Stress also lowers the immune system, making it more likely that you will experience a decline in health.

When the weather is either wet or chilly, many people also experience spikes in FMS. Thus, changes in barometric pressure appear to influence FMS. Just as FMS can be worse in cold weather, it can also worsen when people are in the heat and humidity. Research by the National Fibromyalgia Association showed that people with FMS tended to have worse pain and stiffness during periods of changing weather. People with fibromyalgia may notice that on rainy days they have more problems, or when Autumn comes, their pain levels might increase.

Furthermore, physical and emotional trauma can both cause an increase in the severity of symptoms. Research has found that people with post-traumatic stress disorder (PTSD) are more likely to develop fibromyalgia. If you have gone through something traumatic, your body could feel increased pain levels and tiredness that can negatively impact your ability to function.

Illness also makes FMS worse, and this can also be one of the triggers that causes its onset. Doctors have linked several conditions to FMS, but any illness could potentially trigger it. The flu is one of the most studied diseases that could impact FMS. Other ones that experts have connected to FMS are pneumonia and the Epstein-Barr virus. Bacteria, like shigella and salmonella, can lead to GI issues that result in increased odds of fibromyalgia. Beyond being causal, these illnesses can make it harder for you to manage your pain, and they can worsen the symptoms that you already have.

Too much exercise can also trigger fibromyalgia symptoms. If you exercise too much, you may increase the stress on your body to the point where FMS develops. Exercise is excellent for you. It makes you stronger and healthier, but if you do it in excess, particularly if you have a predisposition for fibromyalgia, it can be problematic.

The causes of fibromyalgia are mostly unknown, so hopefully, increased research will shed some light on this misunderstood condition in the coming years. From the evidence we do have, we can determine that certain things can worsen FMS. This can be highly individualistic, so be sure to pay attention to what triggers symptoms for you personally.

Chapter 2: Signs and Symptoms

Who Fibromyalgia Impacts

You may be surprised by the demographics of people who doctors diagnose with fibromyalgia. Based on what you know, you may guess that fibromyalgia often impacts people of middle age, but it also frequently affects younger people. The exact statistics of fibromyalgia are hard to gather because of how difficult this condition is to diagnose. If there were better diagnostic tests, the understanding of those who fibromyalgia impacts would be much more extensive.

Fibromyalgia can impact people of both genders, but it most common among women, who experience the condition much more often than men. For unknown reasons, some of which may have to do with diagnostic practices, the rates of fibromyalgia among women are steep. Currently, women make up around 90% of the people who are diagnosed with fibromyalgia. Some researchers believe that the high rates of fibromyalgia among women could be hormone related. When they menstruate, many women experience increased symptoms, which could suggest that hormonal factors are triggering the condition.

Doctors diagnosis FMS across many different age groups, but there are certain ages that people tend to develop it more often. Generally, doctors diagnose fibromyalgia in people who are between the ages of twenty to fifty-five. Additional researcher suggests that the bulk of those patients are between thirty-five and forty-five. While most patients experience fibromyalgia at middle-age, these numbers could be skewed by how hard the disorder is to diagnose. Thus, many people may not get a diagnosis until they have already been in pain for years.

No matter what demographic you belong to, you can have fibromyalgia despite what the statistics might suggest. If you are a man who thinks that you may have fibromyalgia, or you are older or younger than the average ages that people get diagnosed, still get checked out and bring your concerns up with your doctor if you're experiencing symptoms. The earlier you can receive a diagnosis and begin treatment, the better your health outcomes and quality of life will be in the long run.

Major Symptoms

Some symptoms stand out as the primary symptoms of fibromyalgia. These symptoms are the ones that most people with fibromyalgia will experience. However, even if you don't have all of these, it is always worth seeking the opinion of a professional because, as is emphasized throughout this book, finding information and facilitating communication with your doctor is imperative.

Pain across your body is the most notable sign of fibromyalgia. When you have fibromyalgia, your pain won't just be limited to one part of your body. You'll usually have several tender points in locations such as your knees, hips, chest, neck, and shoulders. People with fibromyalgia will often ache in several of these points, which can make it hard to feel comfortable. While the pain isn't always sharp, the achiness can be draining, and it can worsen the sleep issues that are often part of fibromyalgia.

You may also be sensitive to touch. People with fibromyalgia may feel pain even when people just brush them lightly. This symptom is called allodynia. This symptom can mean that simple touches like a shoulder rub or a hand on the shoulder can result in extreme pain. Thus, if you know someone with fibromyalgia, you should be careful about where and when you touch them.

Some people may even be sensitive to other senses as well, such as smells, because of their fibromyalgia. This sensitivity can be true for any other of your senses because fibromyalgia can affect the way your body perceives information. In ordinary life, people have a lot of sensations that their brains have to process, and people with fibromyalgia may become overwhelmed trying to process all the senses around them, which can result in their bodies misfiring signals and causing pain in these instances.

Stiffness is another standard symptom of fibromyalgia. Many people will feel stiffness in areas of their bodies that are most impacted by the disorder, such as in the knees, hips, elbows, and neck. This stiffness is often spurred by remaining in one position for an extended period of time. Many people with fibromyalgia will be stiff when they first get up in the morning, and sometimes, this stiffness will cause painful muscle spasms. This stiffness is one of the most challenging symptoms to deal with, but once you have identified it as a problem, there are adjustments you can make to feel better. Medication and physical therapy have both been shown to help people who experience stiffness related to fibromyalgia.

It is usual for people with fibromyalgia to experience brain fog, which is sometimes called fibrofog. Cognitive issues associated with fibromyalgia could make it hard for you to think clearly, even when doing simple tasks.

Sleep disorders are incredibly typical for people with fibromyalgia. Based on research, around ninety percent of people with fibromyalgia experience sleep disturbances. Many people with fibromyalgia may get to sleep, but they don't have a restful sleep, so they aren't able to drift into a deep sleep that leaves them feeling restored. Some people may have trouble sleeping at all, and the pain may make it hard for them to fall asleep, or they may have general fibromyalgia induced insomnia. Once they get to sleep, they may wake up frequently and never make it all the way through the night without waking up. This sleep dysfunction makes it hard to function or think clearly (which could be a factor in fibrofog). It can also lead to extensive fatigue or worsen existing fatigue.

Fatigue is associated with sleep disorders, and it can be caused by the sleep problems that are common among people with fibromyalgia, but it can also occur on its own. Some people with FMS will feel fatigued even when they get ample sleep. While this fatigue can be mild and be the feeling of being just a little tired, it can also be more intense. Some people with fibromyalgia will feel so tired that they'll feel entirely wiped - like you are when you have the flu. This fatigue can make it hard to do tasks like getting exercise, or even simply getting out of bed.

Headaches are also common among people with fibromyalgia. As with fatigue, the headaches can vary in range. Many of these headaches are associated with a stiff neck or shoulders that can radiate up into the head. They can also be induced by the stress of the illness or anxiety. Some people with fibromyalgia will experience migraines, which can make them physically sick.

These symptoms are just a few of the primary symptoms that people with fibromyalgia face. The more symptoms people have, the harder it can be to manage them as these symptoms often compound on one another.

Corresponding Symptoms

In addition to the primary symptoms, some people experience other symptoms that have been attributed to, or worsened by, fibromyalgia.

Irritable bowel syndrome (IBS) can co-occur with fibromyalgia, and the IBS may worsen because of the fibromyalgia. IBS is a condition that can cause constipation, diarrhea, or pain during, or after, bowel movements.

Women may experience worsened periods that are more painful. It's normal for women to have heavier or more painful periods when they have fibromyalgia, and this could be related to hormone dysfunction.

You may feel dizzy or unsteady on your feet. People with fibromyalgia may feel like they can't walk easily or have increased rates of vertigo.

Fibromyalgia can also make you feel too hot or too cold. People with fibromyalgia may have issues with both hot flashes and feeling too cold. This symptom, particularly hot flashes, is one that women often link to menopause, but can be worsened by fibromyalgia.

You may feel a pins and needles sensation in your body if you have fibromyalgia, which is called paresthesia. This symptom impacts twenty-five percent of people with fibromyalgia, and it is usually transient rather than permanent. Thus, while it can feel scary, the sensation most often goes away. Paresthesia most commonly occurs in your extremities, but some people will experience it in other places on their bodies. People with this symptom may worry that they have a neurological disorder (like multiple sclerosis), but that is not always the case. Aside from FMS, it is sometimes caused by high blood pressure, diabetes, a compressed nerve, or infection, which are all avenues to rule out if you have this symptom with few others.

People with fibromyalgia have increased odds of having restless leg syndrome. Restless leg syndrome is a condition that makes people feel an unexplainable urge to keep moving their legs. One-third of people with fibromyalgia will have this condition, compared to just three percent of the population who do not have fibromyalgia.

Some people with fibromyalgia may also experience mental health issues. When you face chronic pain, your mental health may suffer. Problems like depression and anxiety are common among people with fibromyalgia (and there can be an overlap of symptoms), so you can't just look at your physical symptoms, but also must look at your emotional ones as well.

The symptoms associated with fibromyalgia is a long list, but you don't have to experience all of them to have this condition. Many people will encounter different symptoms during different parts of their lives. As you go forward, your symptoms can easily change, and they might become worse or better. Fibromyalgia is dynamic, so what you are experiencing now won't always be what you experience in the future.

Questions to Ask Yourself

This list of questions can help you figure out if you may be experiencing fibromyalgia. Of course, you should always seek the help of a doctor to verify your concerns and ensure that nothing else is wrong, but these questions can give you some insight. If you aren't sure about any of the answers, take some time - a week or so - to contemplate your symptoms and observe how your body feels.

How severe is your pain? Please note that intensity doesn't indicate whether you need medical help or not. If you feel chronic pain at all, that's always a symptom that something is not right, and you need to figure out what that something is. With that in mind, be honest about your pain. Don't try to act tough or underplay what you are feeling, and don't try to make it sound worse than it is to validate it.

Is your pain generalized or targeted? Do you have pain in just one area, or do you have it in several parts of your body? If you feel pain in only one place, you probably do not have fibromyalgia, which is characterized by chronic and widespread pain. If you do not feel widespread pain, you may need to start looking at other explanations for the pain you are feeling.

How long has your pain occurred? Try to remember when you first started experiencing widespread pain. It may take you a while to remember, and you probably won't be able to pinpoint the specific day, but if you have been feeling pain for at least three months, that could be an indicator that you have FMS.

Have you been checked for other conditions? Many conditions can have the same, or similar symptoms as fibromyalgia. Your doctor needs to rule out any other medical conditions before you can be officially diagnosed with FMS. Because there are so many different conditions that fibromyalgia can look like, fibromyalgia is frequently underdiagnosed. It takes a lot of testing for a doctor to rule everything out and ensure that there's no better explanation for your symptoms.

Some conditions that often look like fibromyalgia are thyroid problems, lupus, chronic fatigue syndrome, multiple sclerosis, diabetes, rheumatoid arthritis, anemia, and polymyalgia rheumatica.

Do certain activities make your symptoms worse? Think long and hard about this question. Keep track of the times when your symptoms are most severe. Try to find out if any patterns exist around when you experience symptoms. People with fibromyalgia often have specific activities that make their pain worse. If you can figure out key patterns, you'll be able to avoid or modify certain behaviors to lessen the severity of your symptoms.

How does your pain feel? Is it sharp, dull, or throbbing? While none of these pains will say whether you have fibromyalgia or not, usually, people with fibromyalgia feel aching all over with some sharper pains sporadically.

Answering these questions honestly can help you prepare for your doctor's visit and allow them to more accurately determine if you do in fact have fibromyalgia. The more you understand about how you are feeling, the easier it will be to describe your symptoms to others. Beyond just your doctor, you'll want to inform other significant people in your life. Most of all, you'll want to keep yourself informed. It is a great idea to keep a journal of all your symptoms and track how you are feeling on any given day. By doing this, you can start to identify patterns and will be able to better understand what activities, foods, or external events trigger your symptoms.

Chapter 3: Diagnosis

Diagnostic Criteria

There is no official test for fibromyalgia. While doctors have various methods that they can use to see if you might have FMS, you cannot be one hundred percent sure. If a doctor gives a diagnosis and it doesn't feel right, accept it tentatively until you can further confirm that diagnosis through experience, or you can explain it via new information that you have in the future. It is incredibly difficult when so many conditions may look a whole lot like fibromyalgia.

First, doctors generally like to do blood work and conduct a physical examination to rule out other conditions. They may have you do some further tests if they think you may have conditions not related to fibromyalgia. If something comes back on those initial tests, they might attribute your symptoms to another ailment, but that doesn't mean you don't also have fibromyalgia. When your doctor treats you for that other condition, see if your symptoms improve. If they do not improve after several months, you could still also have fibromyalgia, and you'll want to follow up with your doctor about your concerns.

There are certain factors that a doctor can use to determine if you likely have fibromyalgia. These factors can suggest that you probably have fibromyalgia even if they can't prove it diagnostically. Most doctors will use the following methods, or some very similar ones, to gauge your pain levels.

The first criterion is that on the widespread pain index (WPI) patients score over a seven, and that on the symptom severity scale (SSS), they should get over a five. If they get a score equal to or greater than nine on the SSS, they only need a score of at least four on the WPI. Don't worry about whether or not you meet this criterion right away. Your doctor will ask you questions and use your responses to determine how to proceed and rank your WPI and SSS levels. These scales seem more intimidating than they are. Due to its subjective nature, pain cannot be classified fully by a scale, but be honest with your doctor and you will get the most accurate results possible.

Doctors will also check that patients have pain in at least four of the five regions of the body. Doctors often check specific points on the body to see if they are sensitive and add up the number of these areas to determine if you have fibromyalgia. The tender points for fibromyalgia are in various locations of your body, such as your shoulders, hips, neck, elbows, chest, and knees. In these six areas, there are several points that your doctor can press and will ask you to report your pain levels in those areas.

Your doctor will also ask you how long you have had pain at the current level. You will need to have experienced a comparable pain level for a least three months to be diagnosed with fibromyalgia. However, remember that a myriad of other chronic conditions could also be causing this pain. Pain is a normal part of life, but when you experience it chronically, that's when you know something more serious is occurring.

Diagnostic Issues

There are several issues that people experience when dealing with fibromyalgia and getting treatment. Unfortunately, fibromyalgia is one of the conditions that have a lot of diagnostic issues. The symptoms are just general enough that you can do a quick google search and have hundreds of diseases pop up. With all this uncertainty, it can be distressing for people who have, or think they have, FMS. You may feel that you can never trust a diagnosis, and to some extent, there will always be diagnostic mishaps until we know more about fibromyalgia and related conditions. Nevertheless, make the best with the information you have and listen to your doctor. If you aren't convinced by your doctor's initial diagnosis, don't be afraid to seek a second opinion.

Many people don't realize that they have fibromyalgia. One reason for this is that people are diagnosed with fibromyalgia in middle-age. Thus, they commonly think that the aches and pains they feel are just signs that they're getting older. They might attribute their fatigue to being so busy, possibly having children to look after, and they believe the aches are from their age catching up with them. It's imperative that you take your pain seriously. Maybe it can be attributed to old age, but you don't know until you dig deeper.

The diagnostic criteria make it hard to distinguish fibromyalgia from other conditions, even for doctors who are incredibly knowledgeable about it. As you already know, it can be hard to pinpoint what illness you have when you tell your doctor that you have chronic pain. Even experienced doctors can give you an inadvertently wrong diagnosis. Often, your doctor is not to blame for this mistake, but you need to push your doctor to reevaluate if you think that something is not right with your diagnosis.

Symptoms can be challenging for people to clearly identify at first. This challenge is partially because the symptoms can seem mild at first. For a while, the symptoms can be dull before growing, so people don't notice the pain until it's become incredibly bad. The ache creeps upon them, and before they know it, they are hurting as they do relatively basic things. Not all symptoms will hit full force at once, and you won't necessarily have all the classic signs of FMS, so be more mindful of your body and the changes it endures to keep track of your pain.

How to Find Help

If you think you might have fibromyalgia, you need to seek the advice of a doctor. You cannot get yourself better on your own. There are steps that you can take to improve your pain on your own, but without a diagnosis, you cannot be sure what you need to fix. Thus, before you apply any of the tips in this book on yourself, you need to find help, and this help can come in a myriad of ways. The goal is to find a doctor or a medical team who can accurately diagnose you, and provide treatment options.

The first step is to find a doctor who can help you to help yourself. If you'd like, you can start with the physician that you already have. However, you may also like to do some research and seek out a doctor who has experience dealing with fibromyalgia.

If you're looking for an expert, rheumatologists often have strong understanding of fibromyalgia. They generally deal with rheumatic diseases that are related to the ligaments, joints, muscles, and tendons. Thus, they mostly deal with arthritis, but they also are responsible for more than half of all fibromyalgia diagnoses. They can also rule out other similar feeling conditions like various types of arthritis. Rheumatologists are a great starting point, or you can turn to them if your physician doesn't seem to understand fibromyalgia very well. Doctors have different areas of specialty, so it is often best to coordinate your care with doctors who have done some extra study on the specific issues that you face.

Another professional who you can seek out is a physical therapist. Physical therapists often help people with fibromyalgia move their bodies in new ways so that they can ease their pain through movement. Many physical therapists have experience working with people with fibromyalgia, but you'll want to check their credentials and be sure that they know how to help you best. With the help of your medical support team and your physical therapist, you can figure out what kind of physical therapy would benefit you the most. When you find the right exercises for you, physical therapy can shift the way you interact with your body and help you improve your condition in the process.

Getting help is a crucial step in improving your life if you think you have fibromyalgia. You need to find a professional, or a team of professionals, who can help you not only understand what your issue is, but also help you to manage it. While you can do extensive research on treatments and ways to improve your condition on your own, doctors will have unique medical insight and will know your individual requirements in ways that online sources cannot. Remember to never self-diagnose, and if you aren't happy with the treatment that your doctor is providing, never hesitate to get a second opinion.

Chapter 4: Treatment

Knowing your treatment options is one of the best ways to take charge of your health. A fibromyalgia diagnosis does not mean that you won't be able to do any of the things that you love. With treatment, you can manage your symptoms so that they don't have as profound of an impact on you. There are several options that you can choose from, and it's up to you and your doctor to determine what will work best in your particular situation.

Physical Therapy

Beyond pharmaceutical intervention, other treatments are available to you. Physical therapy is one of these additional treatments that can help you move your body in new ways and keep yourself active, even when you are in pain. While you may want to lay down and not move when you are hurting, dormancy can make your condition worse. Many physical therapists have experience with people with fibromyalgia and will be able to show you the best exercises to help with your symptoms.

Physical therapists can give you some insight into how your body works and how to make it move optimally. Most physical therapists will explain not only what exercise you are doing, but they will explain why you are doing it. These explanations will give you an increased understanding of how your body functions. When you have this logical explanation, you can use that information to propel you forward.

Although it may sound counterintuitive, moving your body can actually help to reduce your pain levels. When you keep your body moving, it builds up a tolerance to physical activity. Some of the best activities for fibromyalgia include stretching, light resistance training, and water activities. These activities do not put a lot of pressure on the joints, but they help you expand your range of movement and build functional strength. When you have more strength and flexibility, your body will be able to move more freely.

Don't let your fear of getting hurt keep you away from physical therapy. Many people think that if they go to physical therapy, they will feel more pain, and they will be forced to do things that they aren't physically ready to do. Physical therapists have been trained to push the body, but also to listen to their clients to be sure that they don't take the session too far. Physical therapy exercise can sometimes hurt in the same way that going to the gym hurts, but if you are communicative of your needs and abilities, your physical therapist can do their best to avoid doing damage. Physical therapy has been shown to help people with fibromyalgia, so rest assured that if your physical therapist is familiar with FMS that they will work within the limits of the condition.

Inform your physical therapist how you feel as you go through treatment. If you're having a bad day on the day of your appointment, be upfront about that bad day. Some people like to push through their pain and hide their pain from others, but you shouldn't do so with people who are trying to help you. Physical therapy works best when you are engaged in it, but not overwhelmed by it.

Learn what works best for you. If you find activities that help, focus on those when you are doing your physical therapy. You don't have to work at the same pace every day, either. Slow down when you need to and realign yourself and your needs. Your needs won't always be the same, so work with your physical trainer to figure out what those needs are during each session. Physical therapy can be a great help if you go into it with the right mindset and continue to express your needs and pain levels throughout the process.

Mental Health Treatment

Mental health treatment may seem unrelated to your fibromyalgia, especially if you do not have mental health issues. However, as mentioned earlier, stress is a huge component of fibromyalgia. Working through any and all mental health issues you have, whether you are conscious of them or not, can greatly reduce stress levels.

Some mental health symptoms can also look similar to fibromyalgia. For example, people with depression may also feel tired. Thus, you could have a mental health condition that exacerbates your FMS, and it will be hard to counteract those symptoms unless you address the mental health issues that fuel them, along with the FMS itself.

People with chronic pain have so much to deal with mentally. When you have chronic pain and other negative symptoms that come with FMS, your whole life changes. You have to approach routine tasks in a different way, as these mundane tasks can cause a great deal of pain for an individual with fibromyalgia. Further, a chronic condition can make you feel hopeless. You might think that things will never get better, and this feeling can lead to mental health issues such as depression. Alternatively, you might have pain when you do a particular activity that you love, and you may develop anxiety or irrational fears as a result. FMS can be a traumatizing condition that changes the way you live your life, so it's no wonder that many people who have FMS also develop (or already have) mental health conditions. These conditions need to be addressed because they only serve to make your FMS worse.

Nearly one-third of people with fibromyalgia report having disturbances in their moods. Some researchers believe that those conditions can cause fibromyalgia, while others believe that fibromyalgia causes mental disorders. The truth could also be a combination of both ideas, and fibromyalgia and mental illness could both exacerbate one another.

Cognitive-behavioral therapy is one of the most common drug-free treatments for fibromyalgia. Among all the mental health treatments, a 2010 analysis suggested that CBT was the most effective. Please note that the use of psychological treatments for your condition does not indicate that your condition is not real. Instead, mental treatments are more frequently being found to help people change their cognitive processes. Some research shows that psychological therapies can make physiological changes in your brain that enable better pain management. CBT is a therapy that challenges the way people think about specific things, and it helps them shift their thinking. For instance, some people may fear that their pain will be awful forever, and they won't have improvement. With CBT, they can learn to become more optimistic and see that pain fluctuates and won't be at its worst forever. In the process, patients can shift the way they think, which will also shift their behaviors.

Seek out a mental health expert if you feel you are more anxious or have a declined mood because of your fibromyalgia. Even if your mental health hasn't declined, it can be a great preventative measure to talk about your feelings before they spiral out of control. If you've just gotten a diagnosis, a mental health professional can help you put your diagnosis into perspective and help you process your feelings in a safe environment. While not everyone has the resources to go to therapy, for some people, it may be necessary or otherwise helpful.

Having a healthy mind frees you to focus on doing things that make you feel better. When you don't have to worry about anxiety, depression, or any other negative mental health outcome, you can spend more time managing your pain and doing activities that help you feel happier overall! It's a win-win scenario that many FMS patients overlook.

Taking care of your mental health is essential for your physical health. If you don't have good mental health, you will not be able to manage your physical symptoms well. The better you feel mentally, the more prepared you will be for the challenges that come with fibromyalgia. While this type of treatment isn't for everyone, it can definitely be beneficial for a lot of FMS patients.

Drugs

Prescription

There are three prescription drugs that the FDA has said are acceptable for the treatment of fibromyalgia. Drug companies have long-established these prescriptions for use with other diseases. Still, in the time since they have existed, they have evolved and have become useful for other conditions like fibromyalgia. Unfortunately, the treatment of fibromyalgia can be tricky, but if you get the right medicine into your system, you can substantially improve your lifestyle and live with less pain. If medication doesn't work at first, don't give up. Sometimes, it takes several weeks or months for medicines to balance with your system thoroughly. Thus, patience and communication with your doctor are the most critical steps that you can take.

Duloxetine, known by the brand name Cymbalta, is an antidepressant that doctors can use to treat fibromyalgia. Milnacipran, more commonly known as Savella, is another antidepressant that doctors sometimes use to treat fibromyalgia. The anti-seizure drug, pregabalin, which goes by the brand name Lyrica, has also been passed by the FDA for treating fibromyalgia symptoms. This medication can be suitable when people have adverse sensory reactions to touch, sounds, or lights. When you start any of these medications, you should monitor any side-effects that you experience, and keep track of your fibromyalgia symptoms to see if the medication is working.

Some doctors may prescribe other medications that the FDA hasn't approved for fibromyalgia specifically. The drugs not being sanctioned does not mean that they are not safe. Mostly, these drugs have not gone through specific trials for fibromyalgia, but medical professionals have discovered that they can be helpful in the treatment of fibromyalgia. If your doctor prescribes these drugs, they will closely monitor you and ensure that you do not have any adverse side effects. Remaining communicative with your treatment team is vital for this reason.

Medication can be an excellent option for people who are severely suffering from fibromyalgia, but some people won't respond well to certain medications. Further, finding the right dosages can take some tweaking. Some people who take antidepressants, for example, may feel mentally worse on a particular drug versus when they take another pill. With a combination of time, and strong communication with your doctors, you can find the right balance for you.

Over-the-counter

Over-the-counter meds can be useful for fibromyalgia, just as prescription ones can be. Acetaminophen is one of the best drugs that you can take for fibromyalgia because of how well it relieves pain. Many people with fibromyalgia also like to take nonsteroidal anti-inflammatory drugs that include naproxen and aspirin. You need to make sure that you talk to your doctor if you want to take these drugs long-term, and you'll want to take them sparingly if you can. Ensure that you do not take more of the drug than your doctor says to take, and also verify that you are not mixing medicines that could be dangerous together. Over-the-counter medications can keep you going when your pain is intense, but there are less traditional pain management methods that you can choose from as well.

Chapter 5: Alternative Medicine

Alternative medicines are great options for people who do not respond well to traditional medicine, or who want to experiment further with their treatment options. You can use these treatments alone, or you can use them with one another, or also with some of the more traditional methods. Adding one or two of these into your lifestyle can transform your relationship with your body. Research has suggested that FMS patients can find success using these methods, but not every technique is for everyone. Track your progress and determine what treatment is right for you.

Acupuncture

Acupuncture is one alternative method that research has suggested improves symptoms among many people with FMS. As a part of traditional Chinese medicine, acupuncture is a practice that has evolved from ancient traditions, and it has long been used to treat a myriad of conditions, many of which are chronic pain diseases. A practitioner will treat specific symptoms that you would like to address when you have a session, rather than managing your fibromyalgia in its totality. If you have a fear of needles, this treatment may not be for you because this treatment is completed by putting needles into your meridians, which are called QI channels, that are located across your body. The needles remain in place for around twenty to forty-five minutes. Beyond needles, acupuncturists may use herbs to promote circulation, or they can utilize electrical pulses to encourage more circulation in your body. Even if you aren't a huge fan of needles, acupuncture could be worth a try as it has been shown to help a large range of people with a wide variety of symptoms.

Massage

If you want something a little less pokey than acupuncture, massage is another helpful method for relieving pain. Not only does this method help you relax, but by releasing the tension from your body, it can also alleviate some of the discomfort that you are feeling. A 2012 Israeli medical review of massage for fibromyalgia showed that several studies supported that massage therapy can be used to reduce the pain and stress that come with FMS. In hospitals, massage is actually the most prevalent alternative therapy that doctors use. When people are massaged, their bodies release endorphins, which are feel-good chemicals that serve as the body's natural version of painkillers. Thus, massage therapy can have similar effects to some over the counter drugs.

Yoga

Yoga helps people focus and work through their pain in a meditative and mindful way. A revolutionary study showed that, in brain imaging, people with fibromyalgia responded to pain in different ways than those who didn't. Their nervous system was more sensitive, which explains the increased pain that they felt. What would be barely noticeable for an average person could be intensely painful for someone with FMS. Through yoga, people can change the way they respond to stress. While fibromyalgia has people react more intensely, yoga calms them and turns down the body's stress response for a while. When you practice yoga, you focus on breathing and poses that allow you to focus your mind on being present in the moment and working through your sensations. Thus, yoga can ease many of the problems that fibromyalgia creates. It teaches you to calm your breathing and take moments of mindfulness throughout the day when you are feeling overwhelmed. Even when you are feeling too tired to do much movement, you can practice breathing and simple poses.

Tai Chi

Research has shown that tai chi can have the same or an even better impact on your fibromyalgia as aerobic exercise, which is known for helping people with fibromyalgia and is one of the first alternative therapies that doctors suggest. Tai chi is another Chinese form of alternative medicine that includes meditative components and calm movements. It is an easy-going activity that gets you moving without overburdening you. By helping you focus on your breathing, tai chi allows you to become more in tune with yourself and to use your mind to reduce your pain. Tai chi combines the forces of mental and bodily power, which can help you if you have mental health issues associated with your fibromyalgia. While the research on the effects of tai chi on fibromyalgia is limited, the studies that have been conducted thus far have shown promising results.

Herbs and Supplements

Several herbal supplements may be able to help you with fibromyalgia. While these herbs aren't a a direct replacement for prescribed or over-the-counter medications, they can help you improve your pain in the long-term, and they are ideal if you are wary of western medicine.

Some people who have fibromyalgia use capsaicin cream, which is a product made from the hot part of chili peppers, to relieve their pain. It can help numb the pain for a while when in a cream form. In one study, people used the cream four times daily, and after one month, their pain levels had decreased.

In Sweden, a study showed that people with low levels of vitamin B12 had unbalanced levels of cerebrospinal fluid, which suggests a link between pain and B12 deficiency. Thus, if you are B12 deficient, supplementing with this nutrient might help you feel less pain.

A vitamin D deficiency can be associated with chronic pain. One study showed that people without sufficient vitamin D had more chronic pain. Further, in another study, people who had generalized chronic pain were deficient in vitamin D ninety-three percent of the time. You should make sure that you have enough vitamin D, and if you don't, you can supplement it. Vitamin D is a common deficiency, so it's certainly something to bring up with your doctor.

Magnesium is in nuts, seeds, and leafy vegetables. Some studies have suggested that if taken over long-term periods, people can reduce their pain. Still, more research needs to be done to see the exact connection between magnesium and FMS.

Herbs like lavender and chamomile can be soothing for people who have fibromyalgia. They can be had in teas, or they can be used in aromatherapy. While they do not necessarily get rid of pain, they can help you calm down enough so that the pain isn't as noticeable.

Herbs and supplements can be fantastic additions to any treatment program, and they can help you find unique ways to fight against your fibromyalgia. Find the nutrients that you have deficiencies in and see if supplementing in these areas can help you to improve your symptoms.

Hypnosis

Hypnosis is another alternative treatment for FMS. Before fibromyalgia was even widely recognized as a medical condition, people have been using hypnotism to deal with chronic pain. While you've probably seen this practice in movies or in a stage show, it is not like the sensationalized version in the media. It is a scientific process that uses the power of your unconscious brain to guide you and help you become more susceptible to suggestions. Please note that it cannot make you do anything that you don't want to do. Instead, hypnosis is a process that puts you into a state that, contrary to popular belief, is not sleeping and is similar (but deeper) than meditation. During this time, you are more focused, which allows you to absorb suggestions.

Studies beginning in the nineties showed that when you add hypnosis to a treatment plan for chronic pain that it can be incredibly useful. Hypnosis has even historically been used in place of anesthesia! Accordingly, further research has shown across six studies that when hypnosis uses guided imagery that it is an effective pain reliever. While hypnosis is not a perfect treatment, many patients do find it helpful. Not everyone can be hypnotized, though, because a small portion of people are resistant to the process. Nevertheless, it is worth a try.

Chapter 6: Tips for Management

Managing your pain and outlook on life requires daily effort. The little management skills that you apply each day will make a profound difference in how you respond to your treatment over the long run. The treatments provided in this book can only take you so far alone, but if you add these tips, you will increase your odds of success in living a life unhindered by fibromyalgia.

Little Acts Make a Huge Difference

You can start with little tasks that will make you feel better. Small actions add up to create massive results, so don't underestimate the power of doing what you can rather than trying to solve every problem at once. Overwhelming yourself will only make it harder to have success in your treatment management, so take it easy on yourself and begin by changing just a few small parts of your life. As you get used to the changes, you can add more and expand your treatment goals.

Taking a warm bath is one great tactic to ease some of your pain. The hot water can be fantastic for your aching body, and a relaxing bath can also reduce the tension you feel from other parts of your life. This action is one of the simplest things that you can do to deal with pain, particularly if you use Epsom salts. Epsom salts are rich in magnesium, which as mentioned before, can assist in easing fibromyalgia symptoms. You can also try using heating pads or heated blankets to give your body some warmth, which can be comforting and make you feel better all around.

Aim to do several tasks a day, even if they are little ones. You don't need to do everything on your list to feel good, but you do need to remain active and not give up on yourself.

Complete tasks incrementally rather than trying to do everything at once. The truth is that you aren't always going to have the energy to do everything at once. For example, completing tasks around the house can be daunting. You may try to set aside a whole day to clean your house, and you'll find yourself feeling incredibly achy and exhausted after, or while, you are cleaning. The exertion of cleaning can completely drain you, which makes your FMS worse than it was before, and this exertion does not promote long-term improvement. If this sounds familiar, you can try breaking up your cleaning into smaller, individual tasks, rather than trying to do everything at once.

Distractions can make a big difference when your symptoms flare up. If you need to binge-watch a TV show to keep your mind off your pain, do it. Sometimes, you just need something mindless to get your mind away from the pain, and you shouldn't feel guilty for needing that.

When you feel energized, make good use of that energy while you have it. It's good to use times when you are feeling good to your advantage but, do be careful not to overexert yourself. Be mindful of your energy levels and how you are feeling and learn your limits through experimentation. The longer you manage your pain, the more you'll start to see trends and understand your limitations. Knowing how much you can do may be hard now, but over time you will gain a better understanding of just how far you can safely push yourself.

Experimenting with your treatment plan is another excellent way to ensure you stay as pain-free as you can. When one thing doesn't work, try another combination. Remember, to stay in contact with your doctor and get their approval before making any changes to your treatment plan. Give new treatments some time – at least a few weeks. However, if you aren't seeing any results after a few weeks or a couple of months, consider mixing up your treatment.

Remember to have gratitude. When you are feeling pain, finding things to be grateful for can put you in a better mental space. Think about what you are lucky to have and think about all the wonderful things your body can do, even if it has limitations. Learn to be thankful for still being alive and being given a chance to make the best of your life. There's much more to be glad for than there is to be unhappy about, and by focusing on those things, you can shift your mind from the pain.

Be selfish, sometimes. There will be times when you have to miss events or not do certain things with loved ones for the sake of your own well-being, and that's okay. You don't need to risk your health to please other people. You'll want to do certain things, and you won't be able to do them without making your health worse, so remain conscious of what future consequences your actions may have. Remember that you cannot help people if you do not first help yourself.

You don't have to change your whole life overnight to feel better. Taking small steps to deal with fibromyalgia can make a huge difference. These small steps will compound over time, and before you know it you will be in a much better space both physically and mentally.

Lifestyle Habits

A few lifestyle changes can make a massive impact on your fibromyalgia symptoms. When you take care of yourself, you're in a better place to fight your symptoms and work on improving them. These lifestyle changes will work to reduce your stress, both physical and mental.

Exercise is one of the best habits that you can develop. Aerobic activity is one of the most popular alternative treatments that doctors suggest. While exercise doesn't seem appealing when you are in pain, putting in just a few minutes a day can transform your health. Additionally, exercise releases endorphins, which make you feel good and can act in the same way as pain killers. Thus, while it can be hard to find the motivation to get active, being active will ultimately make you feel better. Once again, start slow and don't overexert yourself. Consulting with a physical therapist is a great idea when you're first trying to develop an exercise routine that works for you.

Nutrition is another critical lifestyle component. If you don't have a balanced, healthy diet, your body will be prone to more pain. When you eat well, your body can deal with pain better. Eat a variety of foods, making sure that you include a lot of vegetables in your diet. You should also aim to limit your sugar intake, as studies have shown that excess sugar can make pain worse in people with fibromyalgia.

You need to learn to manage your stress. Because of the theoretical connections of FMS with your nervous system response, when you feel stressed, your body is more likely to trigger pain signals. You'll feel that you are in a dire situation, even if you are not. Destressing isn't always an easy task, but when you're stressed, you're more likely to experience fibromyalgia symptoms.

Get your sleep. While it may be hard to sleep because of your condition, the body needs adequate sleep to repair itself and function optimally. While you can't always control your sleep, and you may have insomnia or other sleep issues, there are steps you can take to improve your chances of getting quality sleep. Before bed, for instance, you should limit your technology use because blue light can make it hard to sleep. Further, it would help if you took the time to relax and clear your mind prior to going to bed. You might like to drink a cup of decaffeinated tea before bed or relax in a room with some calming essential oils.

Most importantly, you need to make time for sleep. Never use the excuse that you are too busy to sleep! You are too busy not to sleep. Sacrificing sleep will make you more exhausted, and it will only worsen your FMS symptoms.

Dive into things that you make you feel fulfilled, and if something makes you feel like you have a purpose and energizes you, dive into that activity. Passions make you feel alive, and they can boost your energy and give you a great distraction that makes you forget about your pain for a while.

Work less and play more, when possible. Sometimes, you don't have much choice in your work schedule, but during your free time, let your time be entirely free. Don't continually check your work email when you're at dinner, and don't rearrange your life around your work. As stated several times already, stress plays a large role in the severity of fibromyalgia symptoms. Switching off and taking time to relax needs to be a priority in your life if you wish to improve your FMS.

Social Circumstances

Your social life can play a large role in how you feel both mentally and physically. People are not lone wolfs, and even introverts need some level of human connection. Unfortunately, chronic illness can make it go hard to go out into the world and be social. Do your best to communicate with friends and family about your symptoms, and organize social activities that you can participate in without worrying that they will be too physically challenging for you.

At the same time, when other people drain you, limit your interactions with them. It's okay to say no to invitations or express that you need time to yourself. You don't always have to be social. You will sometimes want time alone to think or rest, and that's healthy. Find the balance that works for you.

Don't compare yourself to people who don't have FMS. Comparison only serves to make you feel inadequate. When you compare yourself to other people, you make judgments about yourself. These judgments don't help you, and they can put you in a worse mental state than you were to begin with.

Spiritual Avenues

While not everyone is spiritual, spirituality can be a source of strength for many people. If you are spiritual, you can use your spirituality or your religion to motivate you to keep going and help you fight through your symptoms. Being spiritual doesn't mean that you need to be religious, so however you practice spirituality, incorporate that into your process of self-help. If you don't believe in anything spiritual, you might instead like to think about your greater purpose.

Think of your higher power, if you recognize one. It doesn't have to be God or another deity. It can be anything that gives you purpose and overarches your value system, making you want to do better as a human being. For example, if you love nature and want to preserve it, your higher power may be nature. Higher powers make you feel less alone, and they show that while there's so much that's out of your control, you are in control of what you focus on.

Always remind yourself of all the things in life that give you purpose. These are the things that will keep you going through the most challenging parts of your illness, and they will remind you that there's so much more to you than your symptoms.

Getting Creative

Creativity is an excellent way to manage pain. Finding creative outlets to help keep your mind and body busy is vital for your mental and physical well-being. Creative endeavor is also a fantastic way to work through stress.

There are so many ways to be creative. One of the best ways is to journal. Journals allow you to document your feelings and experiences, which can help you track the changes you are facing and monitor yourself. Other creative endeavors like creative writing, model building, and art are all great options. Creative endeavors aren't about how good you are at them. They are about expression and enjoyment, so find that expression and enjoyment, regardless of how great (or not so great) your artwork looks.

Conclusion

Thank you for making it through to the end of this book. I hope that it was enlightening and could provide you with some more information about fibromyalgia, and how it can be managed and improved.

Remember to never self-diagnose, and instead consult with a doctor if after reading this book you feel as though you may have fibromyalgia.

Strive to create a treatment plan that works for you, and don't hesitate to experiment with some of the alternative therapies in conjunction with the pharmaceutical treatments that your doctor may prescribe.

Once again, thanks for choosing this book. I hope you have found it to be helpful, and I wish you the best of luck!

9 781761 035852